WHY YOU SHOULD TAKE A BREAK FROM DRINKING AND HOW TO DO IT

WHY YOU SHOULD TAKE A BREAK FROM DRINKING AND HOW TO DO IT

DAVID DOWNIE

WHY YOU SHOULD TAKE A BREAK FROM DRINKING
AND HOW TO DO IT.

See other books by the Author at his Amazon author page:
www.amazon.com/author/bestsellers

Published by Blue Peg Publishing

If you have purchased the ebook version of this book, then please
consider buying the print version if your family enjoys the ebook.

Contents

ABOUT THE AUTHOR

David Downie is the founder of AustralianBeers.com and the Austraian contributor to the international beer bible *1001 Beers You Must Drink Before You Die*. He was profiled in the book *Three Sheets to the Wind* by leading UK beer expert Pete Brown.

David is also the author of 2 books on contract law and 6 illustrated children's books, some of which have been translated into over 40 languages. He assisted the author of the *Macquarie Book of Slang* with several of its less salubrious definitions.

David has honors degrees in both science and law and is a former Partner at a major Australian law firm.

David has appeared on Sky News and has been quoted by publications including the Australian Financial Review, Business Review Weekly and the Sydney Morning Herald as an expert in law, children's books, beer and Australian culture. The BBC asked to interview him about a light version of VB, but he declined as he refused to drink it (even before he was between drinks).

FAQ – DEFENSIVE DRINKERS READ THIS

Is giving up alcohol for a period for you? If you have made the choice to seek out this book and read this far, then chances are it is. After all, what's the worst thing that can happen? That you take up old habits? Big deal. The potential upside for your life is enormous.

Do I have to be an alcoholic?

Not at all. In fact, if you are an alcoholic then please do me a favour and return this book. Real alcoholics can run into real trouble stopping drinking, even for a limited period. See your doctor. This book is for 'normal' drinkers, even if they like a binge (or two) on the weekends.

Do I have to give up alcohol forever?

No! Unless you want to. Sitting on the balcony at 83 and not having a glass of wine while you are on your last legs sounds pretty grim. You don't have to do this. Read this book and you can have t all.

Will my drinking friends still love me if I stop drinking?

Of course they will. Chances are they will be more curious than critical. Whether or not you still love them once you view them sober is another question.

Do I have to get fit, quit my job or dump my partner?

Not necessarily. Clear Thinking obtained by not drinking gives you the perspective to see your life for what it is. Another happy side effect of not drinking is that you have the time, energy and brain power to use this insight to change things so that your life becomes awesome. Whether or not making a better version of you involves getting fit, quitting your job or dumping your partner will be entirely your decision.

MY STORY AND WHY YOU NEED THIS BOOK

I pounded the paste some more, the wonderful fragrance of chili, garlic and coriander root tickling my nose.

"We need some more galangal", I whispered, with some urgency, to my new girlfriend Jane, who was hovering nearby. Smiling, she grabbed a knife and made out for the garden to harvest some.

"And lemongrass!", I cried after her.

An hour or so later we were eating the most stunning thai curry either of us had ever encountered. No less than 7 of the ingredients for it had been grown in my garden.

It tasted even better because it was lunchtime on a weekday, and all of my old coworkers were no doubt at their desks reading legal contracts.

Three years ago probably wouldn't have been interested in growing that food, or pounding the paste before lunch. I wouldn't have been hung over as such (most days), but I could have been a little flat, perhaps without even realising it. Certainly too flat to enjoy doing the things Jane and I had been doing this week – swimming in waterholes, riding horses, volunteering at a local school and building a food forest in my back yard.

Three years ago I would most likely have been at work too, as a Partner in a massive law firm, and possibly entertaining clients as 'the beer guy', founder of Australia's leading beer website,[1] and contributor to the international book on beer, '1001 Beers You Must Drink Before You Die'.[2]

All lofty and pretty cool stuff. But it didn't involve me not going to work, finding a new girl and moving to a paradise near the beach on the Gold Coast of Australia to make a curry paste from my garden.

That came later.

It came after I gave up alcohol for a year, on a whim, not long after the 1001 beers book was published. After I pushed myself though the physical, social and mental challenges that giving up the grog presented, and ended up with a zen like clarity about my own life and alcohol's effect on it.

I wasn't alone. I sought out like minded men and women who had similar stories and almost to a person they reported back that abstaining had changed them and their lives permanently - for the better. It wasn't that alcohol was killing them (well, most of them), but rather that the cycle of drinking, being hung over or tired and then planning for another drink had stopped them from seeing their lives objectively. From living deliberately.

These Clear Thinkers, as I called them, were not just healthier and happier off the drink, but were actually making *real changes* to the way they lived at a macro level. They

---

[1]   AustralianBeers.com.
[2]   33 beers reviewed thanks very much.

were able to see the woods for the trees, taking take a step back and viewing the world, and themselves, as they truly were – Matrix style.

Some of them, like me, ended up quitting their jobs. Others (like me, for a period) worked out how to do their jobs better to earn more money or take back more time. Some split from their partners and found new love. A select few slept better at night after working out that, as they had suspected, their lives were pretty much in order after all (but thanks for all the extra time!).

Most didn't return to the drink after their time off. At least for now.

As for me... well, I've spent the past three years as a Clear Thinker completely rewriting my life's script. It turns out that my existence as a beer expert and partner in a major law firm wasn't how I wanted to spend my time after all.

My life between drinks is much more exciting than that.

My alcohol chronology

Age 12

Introduced to beer by my 15 year old cousin at the Stradbroke sland pub. Bouncers think about throwing me out for reasons other than my age, but don't. I trade my beer for a chocolate liquor as it tastes funny.

Age 14

Start drinking for real. Friend's 16 year old brother tells me that alcohol "is an acquired taste, but a taste well worth acquiring". As far as I can tell, he's right.[3] I form strong bonds with peers while drinking Jim Beam before moving to beers. My parents think I am having sleepovers and watching videos.

Age 17

Seasoned drinker among the Brisbane pub scene. Fake IDs grant me full access rights, which is just as well as I'm at university man, and going to pubs with your mates is what kids do. It's awesome.

Age 23

Spend a year abroad in Canada working as a tent erector and C++ programmer. Change workmates' lives for the better through drink, but they secretly think I'm an alcoholic. Obviously they have never been to Australia, or the UK for that matter.

Age 24

Return to Australia with an international drinking perspective. Decide to share my new 'knowledge' with the world and form AustralianBeers.com (which I still run, some 14 years later). This in turn introduces me to Australia's top brewers, and their beers. A revolution is happening in Australian brewing, and I have a front row seat.

The Sydney Morning Herald calls me "a dedicated suds swiller, with a genuine appreciation of pub culture". I ask my family to inscribe this on my tombstone when the time comes.

---

[3]   See   http://www.brewsnews.com.au/2011/04/beer-a-taste-worth-acquiring/
for an article written by the 'old me'.

Age 25

Go off the drink for 8 weeks after suffering from work related panic attacks. Promptly get fit, start snorkelling Sydney beaches and lose 8 kg (1.3 stone). Seem more relaxed so start drinking again and replace the beach for the beer garden before regaining the weight.

Age 29

The UK's leading beer expert says in his book on international beer culture that I "love not only beer but the culture that surrounds it and what that culture says about being Australian."[4]

He also says that I thought about beer exactly the same way he did.

This pleases me immensely.

Age 33

Become Partner in Queensland's largest law firm, in part due to being everyone's best mate as I'm a beer guy. I regularly host beer tasting evenings for clients and have at least one long lunch a week. Tasty, although my pants keep shrinking for some reason.

Age 35

I'm asked to represent Australia in the leading international book on beer: *1001 Beers You Must Drink Before You Die*. I

---

[4]   Three Sheets to the Wind by Pete Brown.

see this as equivalent to winning a gold medal at the beer Olympics.

I write 33 beer entries, which on a per capita basis must be up there. It is fun, but hard, thirsty work.

The book is published in many languages around the world and I see it in airports when I travel. The Sydney Morning Herald noted that I had a passion for beer. This also pleases me.

Truth be told though I'm exhausted, and once the massive beer book (my gold medal?) arrives I decide to take 12 months off the drink as an experiment.

Age 38

Still between drinks. Not drinking has given me the ability to sit back and think about my life, which has resulted in me making massive changes, including clearing all my debt. As I write this I'm watching the sun rise over bush land in the Australian Gold Coast hinterland. Kookaburras are making their early morning calls and hunting grubs in my vegetable garden. Most of the fruit trees are sprouting in anticipation of spring.

I won't be going to work today as I threw in my massive job for a better existence. Instead, I'll be going to the beach, which is free.

In my alternative, sliding-doors existence, I wouldn't be writing at this hour (5.30 in the morning). I wouldn't even be here. I would be in the city feeling a little less than optimal (at best), getting up and going in for the slog. Flat. Tired.

Thinking about maybe catching up with a mate for a drink on Thursday night to lie about girls and moan about clients.

You know what I'm talking about. And it doesn't have to be this way.

Not drinking, at least for a while, can help you get your life back to what it should be: off the mindless, drunken treadmill that goes hand in hand with the rat race and into something deliberate and authentic.

Something *you* choose, not the system. Not your booze ridden culture or your mates.

You.

THE GOOD, THE BAD
AND THE UGLY

Ale, man, ale's the stuff to drink
For fellows whom it hurts to think:
Look into the pewter pot
To see the world as the world's not.

A.E. Housman, 1896

Alcohol is, of course, fantastic. Let's get that out of the way up front. I don't buy all that fire-and-brimstone crap.

Drinking is one of life's great pleasures: it's exhilarating; it's sensuous; it's seductive; it eases your worries; it brings people together; it makes you feel good, and, perhaps most important of all, it makes *other* people feel good.[5]

I have written before (back in my drinking days) about how alcohol can be a part of a life well lived, and I truly believe that. There can be sophistication in drinking and a whole heap of fun, which is, after all, a big part of what we hope to get out of life, isn't it. Fun in taste, fun with mates, and even fun in excess.

To be between drinks is not to be down on other drinkers.

---

[5] Admit it. You first kissed your partner drunk didn't you. God knows we have all been there.

So what distinguishes a Clear Thinker from a serious (typical) drinker?

Let's take a look.

D: Social time revolves around having a drink with friends.

CT: Social time revolves around doing extremely cool, high quality things with friends (like white water rafting, writing a movie script or making a curry paste) rather than getting pissed over and over and over and being too tired to do the fun stuff.

D: First thing Saturday morning is not a good time to play with your 3 year old nephew or appreciate the finer qualities of a walk through a beautiful natural setting.

CT: First thing Saturday morning is your favourite time of the week for doing things — because you know you should feel hung over and instead you feel fantastic!

D: Tries to gain courage with the opposite sex by getting drunk and staying out until 3 in the morning.

CT: Quickly learns that all the fun stuff can be done sober and becomes the quickest witted person in the room who can outsmart and outlast anyone (it's almost not fair on the drunks...). In truth though, the inebriated start to become very boring and unattractive after an hour or so and you would prefer to be home by 12 as you're doing something incredibly awesome in the morning (which, unsurprisingly, makes you even more intriguing).

D: Justifies drinking first by reference to friendship/peer bonding, and then if that becomes ridiculous or they come into money, by pretending to be sophisticated (no, I'm not getting pissed, I know all about this vineyard and you're just ignorant).

CT: Knows getting pissed is getting pissed – dress it up all you like. It's still slurping alcohol so you get a buzz. Tasting a fig in your wine won't stop you from getting pissed. In fact, it's the only reason your lizard brain has commanded your conscious brain to drink it. As for your mates, yeah at 17 it makes sense (sort of). At 36 it's getting pathetic (or at the least, tired). There's a spectrum in between.

D: Invariably end up with a beer gut or 'booze tits' (or both) as a combination of the huge amount of empty calories in alcohol, too many dodgy curries/kebabs and too many recovery fry ups. Not to mention a lack of will to exercise after a night out.

CT: Finds the weight falls off you without trying off the drink, and that it also provides an amazing platform to get into a fabulous food and exercise routine that would normally be smashed with a big night out or two. That combined with clearer skin soon gets everyone talking (but ultimately you don't care what they think).

D: If they are honest, discover first that their IQ drops the morning after a few drinks (do you really try and solve complex problems the day after?), and, more disturbingly, that they generally aren't quite as smart as they were when they were 20.

CT: Pleasingly finds that problems get easier to solve after a couple of months off the drink. Is it such a shock that you get smarter after you stop punishing your brain with drink? Hangovers hurt your head for a reason.....

D: Functions as best they can at work, given they aren't quite feeling 100% some days and can't wait to knock the frost off a cold one other days.

CT: Uses a crisper brain to outperform the drinker as well as scheme to achieve considered outcomes. Does the drinker have any considered outcomes in mind?

D: For many, life consists largely of either being drunk, being hung over or planning on being drunk again.[6] Not you? Think about what your social plans are at the moment. How did you spend the last two weeks? What's on your mind?

CT: A zen like clarity descends after 6-12 months off the drink that allows one's life to be seen for what it is, warts and all. Increased intelligence and a greater awareness allow you to make a plan for better things and act on it (using all the time you free up not being drunk or hung over). Meanwhile, your friends get pissed and stay stuck in the rut they probably don't even know they are in.[7]

Of course, you don't need to have a zen like clarity all of the time. Does someone who lives in their perfect house and makes love to their perfect partner every night while living on passive income need zen like clarity? Does it matter he or she is 20 IQ points lower and is a little crabby before 10?

Not really.

But most of us haven't reached nirvana. Becoming a Clear Thinker can help you move in the right direction. And, if your

---

[6]   As well as earning money to pay for the drink and the costs that go with it.
[7]   As the years tick by.

life became wonderful off the drink, would you want to risk losing it all by going back to your old ways?

That would be up to you.

Where you don't want to end up is the dementia unit, as one of our family friends did. Lovely fellow. Really enjoyed his beer. Probably much like some of your friends do, and perhaps even you.

Loved popping off to the pub when he could and having a laugh.

All fun and games in his 20s. Probably slightly less socially acceptable in his 30s and 40s. And completely awful in his 50s, when all that booze and its brain affecting ways hit home and he became so muddled (read: brain damaged) that his family had him committed to a dementia ward.

Horrifying.

He knew he was there alright. He did his best to get out. Applied to court and all the rest of it. But alcohol had transformed him from the person he was at 20, to something less. Something desperate. Something broken.

Eventually he got out, after some years of living in a locked ward. He is in a half way unit now, with other drunks. His family visit him every now and then.

Not often.

That's an extreme story, but it is one of the potential side effects from keeping up the boozing. Another fellow I knew lost his legal career because he urinated on another lawyer's face while he was sleeping on a work retreat (the drinker thought he was in a toilet). We debated whether or not the poor fellow who was rudely awoken should have told HR.

In the end we couldn't blame him.

Anyway, we all know (or should know) that bashing the bottle can lead to early death or diminished quality of life.[8] I knew it back when I was a drinker, and, to be honest, I didn't give a shit. I was (relatively) young. I didn't drink that much.[9]

No, I gave up the drink for 12 months because:

- I was tired of feeling tired and being unfit;
- my gold medal beer book had come out so I was confident nobody could slag me off;
- I was curious about what life would be like off the drink; and
- I had nothing to lose by having some time off. What's the worst that could have happened? I had another drink? Big deal.

It was my choice to take time off the drink. My decision. Of course, it wasn't always easy, because drinking was such a large part of my life and I thought it was brilliant....

---

[8]   In Russia the male life expectancy is only around 60, because they get pissed so much (elsewhere it's in the high 70s). Over 500,000 Russians get killed by too much booze each year.
[9]   Or did I?

17

TAKING A BREAK

So-called pleasures, when they go beyond
a certain limit, are but punishments.

- SENECA (4 B.C.-A.D 65).

So clearly there is an upside to taking a break – if only a short one – from the drink. I've spoken about why I did it, and I am confident that by reading this book you are sufficiently curious about life without booze to put your hand up for a while.

How long you want to be between drinks for is completely up to you. It is an important distinction, I think, to be *between drinks* versus being a *non-drinker*, or worse, a *teetotaler*.[10] Putting my drinker's cap back on (yes it still fits, sort of), a non-drinker brings to mind:

- the old expression *never trust a man who doesn't drink*;
- the bloke who can't pick up a girl to save himself;
- the girl who is 26 and has never had sex; and
- overall, someone who is *a bit strange*.

Naturally, you are none of those things, and presumably don't want to be seen by anyone as such. And in any event you are not swearing never to have a drink again – I haven't, why would you, and in doing so you are setting yourself up for failure and then some.

---

[10]   Although I think those last two are the same thing

No, drinking isn't bad remember.[11] Drinking is awesome.[12] But some people (some *smart* people) take a step back once in a while and see for themselves if they are now at a stage in their lives where not drinking is even more awesome.

If it isn't, you can just go back to your old ways.

The greater the time you take off the drink the more likely you are to be able to make an informed decision as to whether or not your life is better off the drink than not.

Taking a day off the drink is not really going to prove anything. I'm not talking true blue alcoholics here (and if that's you, see your doctor), but if you are spending your life having a drink with the boys or girls, then having a day off to recover before jumping back into it, then that's about as bad a cycle as it gets.

You're basically drinking all the time.

It all depends on you and your level of (social and physical) dependency on the stuff but I think really to get some sense of the possible you should try and put your hand up for a month. Otherwise you'll be suffering withdrawal symptoms the whole time you are off.

If that seems impossible then that's fine too. Try a night or two. Stretch your AFDs (alcohol free days) out to a week, then two. It really has to be something you want to do for yourself, so there aren't any rules here. There is no right or wrong. But if you want to be able to make an informed choice as to

---

[11]   Let's keep with this until you gain perspective at least....
[12]   I'll never disagree with this!

your quality of life, then you need to give yourself a decent amount of time off the sauce.

Of course, while some may glimpse life on other side after a month or so, to give yourself the best chance of developing the perspective we have been talking about – of you becoming a Clear Thinker – then you need to consider at least 6 months off the drink.

In my case, I think I needed the twelve months I committed to as alcohol was so entrenched in my life. Socially, of course, that was how I interacted with my mates. But professionally, as a Partner in a law firm, and a lawyer before that, I was expected to drink with clients at least twice a week.[13]

On top of that I had the beer guy reputation with the website and the book. Everyone wants to have a drink with the beer guy. And of course I had to drink the free samples I was regularly sent to keep up to date with things.

Of course.

So I needed the full 12 months. But you might not. And it could seem too full on, in which case start small. You can always extend the experiment if seems to be going well. Or run another one later on.

Once you have committed to a period off the drink then you are away!

---

[13] Or so I thought. This was most likely a self justification. People who want to drink find excuses to drink. All of a sudden it just seems like a good idea to catch up with an old mate? Probably it's the lizard brain complaining it's thirsty.

ACTIONS

1. Ask yourself if you are curious about gaining some perspective off the drink to realign your priorities and create a better version of yourself.
2. Pick a time to take off the drink, being a minimum of a month and maximum of a year (6 months or more is ideal).

FIRST STEPS

Unless you are hopeless recluse then the first thing you should do is tell everyone you can about your decision to take some time off the drink. Then at the least it's embarrassing if you back down.

You are of course likely to be met with a range of responses. Some people will be supportive. Others curious. Others incredulous. And of course some dickheads will try and stop you.

In my case I had well meaning but honestly pretty thick people telling me I couldn't start this week because the group Christmas party was on. But that's the point isn't it — there is always something on. If there wasn't always something on, then you wouldn't need to give it a rest, would you.

The deniers will just tell you flat out you can't do it. They may even laugh at the thought. Well, you can show them. The fact they have reacted so does tell you something about how people perceive you though.

You may even be unlucky enough to encounter hostility. *It is just not British* to be off the drink. *What would the diggers think?*

That is of course bullshit. Generally the greater the reaction the more likely it is the person reacting has their own issues to deal with.

It's helpful to keep a diary from the beginning. Some people keep anonymous blogs and obtain support by their readers. Really though the writing is for your own benefit, and will allow you to track how you are going, vent your frustrations and so on. It might also be useful for you to read what other people have gone through.

Physical reactions

*Wine drunk to excess affects the body
in a certain way*

Hippocrates, circa 400 BC

You might think you are not physically addicted to the drink, but your body is likely to disagree. If you think about it, your body freaks out if it doesn't get caffine for a couple of days, and drink s a much more powerful drug than that.

Alcoholics of course are in for a world of pain, and need medical supervision.

As for me, I was surprised about the extent of the physical effects of stopping, which consisted first up of me overreacting to situations, snapping at people who didn't deserve it, and generally being more unpleasant than I normally am.

Marvellous.

I also developed a stinking headache to go with it, which I promptly attacked with painkillers. More disturbingly, for a bloke who didn't have a problem, was that on at least one occasion I found myself light headed, which turned out to be due to a fluctuation in blood pressure brought about by not being on the drink.

How crazy is that?

Nothing serious, in my case. There was one night when I found myself scratching my arms, like a recovering addict, but surely that had nothing to do with it....

It isn't all bad though. The minor symptoms are much easier to deal with than a bad hangover and generally last less than 10 days.[14] More excitingly, I started noticing some positives from not imbibing within the same period.

First up, my face was less puffy and started to look much clearer. Second, I started sleeping like a baby – waking fully rested. Third was my fitness levels improved out of sight – my training companion on the weekend after the big decision was confused and said I was like a different person (I hadn't mentioned I was off the sauce).

To top it off I started getting comments I was looking better almost immediately.

All fabulous, and this was just the beginning.

---

[14] If you get the shakes or have anything else happen that is any way disturbing then you've underestimated your dependency on the stuff and need to see your doctor quick smart. They can help you get through this without making it any more difficult than it has to be.

FIRST TIME AMONG DRINKERS

Imagine the drunken man's behaviour
extended over several days: would you not
hesitate to think him out of his mind?

- SENECA (4 B.C.-A.D 65).

Not being an alcoholic means that the physical challenge is the least of it - your body feels better off the drink, after all. The real tests come in the form of cultural, social and environmental challenges, all of which are very real.

Your first challenge is likely to be the first time you have to spend time with drinkers. It goes without saying that initially you should try and avoid situations you strongly associate with drinking — like the damn pub! You will get there eventually but to rock on up with your mates the day after you make a decision is pure madness, and setting yourself up for failure.

Eventually though, you will have to spend an evening or an afternoon with people who are on the sauce, having the time of their lives.

Nothing better really is there, than an ice cold beer on a lazy summer day in the sun.......

See, that's the trap. Drinking is awesome, and that siren call can be your undoing. Especially since you are essentially still the addicted and conditioned person you were when you made the decision to go cold turkey for a while.

But, eventually it will happen. In my case it was a group Christmas dinner (yes, the one I was warned about), in the fanciest restaurant in town. No expense spared. Beautiful wines, beers, liquors – you name it, it was there, it was free, and everyone was getting on it.

Unquestionably, in the beginning, you will feel like you are missing out. You *are* missing out, at least in your mind.[15] You will be acutely aware of what's ordered and who gets what and that YOU MISS OUT. This will be made worse by other people constantly trying to give you a drink, or, if they are aware of your ambition, possibly urging you to have 'just one'.

Be strong. If you have told them what you are up to, perhaps just say no I'm taking a spell off the booze (ie you are still a drinker but are just between drinks). Or if you don't want to have the same conversation (and debate) over and over you can perhaps say you are driving or are on medication that means you can't drink.

You may feel at times that you are causing trouble, or that people are thinking less of you because of your decision. But the truth is, like almost every other aspect of your life, nobody cares – just as you wouldn't care if your mate had a night off the drink for some reason. You would just carry on and get pissed like you always do, but not really give a shit, because it's all about you.

Same with them.

The feeling of missing out will peak in the first hour. After that time, you will notice things about drinkers you have never

---

[15] Truth is, by the time you become a Clear Thinker, you won't think you're missing out. 12 months into my own little adventure, I didn't even notice other people drinking, 99 times out of 100.

noticed before. Think of it as a little experiment. While you have always been pleased to find you got wittier and better looking the more you drank, you will find to your surprise that is not true of others.

The laughter will start to get a little unhinged. Stories will be told and retold. As the night goes on confidence will rise in the most unlikely of people, and fat blokes in suits will take to the dance floor certain that their big city job will finally prove irresistible to the hot 19 year old in the short skirt.[16]

Inevitably the wild eyes and blurred words will appear, along with the shots. Advice will be given that is considered profound but is in fact meaningless. People will spit in your face without knowing it. They look terrible. They act appallingly. It is nothing like you recall.

It is disgusting and disturbing at the same time. If you think about it – and you will – you might even come to the realisation that all of those amazing fabulous nights you have had with the guys and girls over the years have been equally as messy, and not in a good way. You've just been another one of these drunken fools thinking they are top of the pops but who are really just pissing away their time and money. You might even recall particular nights out you have had with a touch more shame than you used to.[17]

---

[16] It won't.

[17] You don't want to dwell on the past. I felt a bit sick when I recalled the hundreds of nights I drunkenly pushed premium beer on people as though I was some sort of enlightened saviour. They needed saving all right. From the grog monster trying to force them to drink more in the name of sophistication...

Eventually the witching hour will be upon you. That is not a good time for a sober person to be out. The fat guys in the suits are now sitting in the corner, taking advantage of their girth to have an extra few pints by themselves to drown their sorrows. The girl in the short skirt, swaying with the biggest fuckwit in the room on the dance floor, is only 6 hours away from her walk of shame.

Anyone left standing by the bar is speaking in tongues. None of it makes any sense at all, and in fact is a bit scary.

You certainly don't feel you are missing out if you survive this long.

If you crack, and have a drink or 20, it's no big deal. There is no exam or confession to make in front of a room full of people with sunken eyes. Just reconsider your options the next day.

If you don't crack, the morning will be a source of wonder for you. You'll wake and have the incredible feeling of knowing that you should be hung over, but aren't. That's one of the best things to come out of this experiment. I urge you to take advantage of it by doing something you would never do hung over: go for a walk or a run, visit your mother, play with some children.

You will know what it is you would be most unlikely to do hungover - do it!

I find time in nature to be the most rewarding, as there is no way you can appreciate the subtle beauty in life with a hangover. The amazing becomes the annoying, and the only thing appreciated is a fry up and painkiller.

ACTIONS

1. When inevitably faced with drinkers, enjoy studying their deterioration – treat it as an experiment
2. Do something awesome when you would normally be hungover – create your own 'Sliding Doors' moment.

KEEPING
THE FAITH

*Oh, that men should put an enemy in their mouths to steal
away their brains! That we should, with joy, pleasance
revel and applause, transform ourselves into beasts!*

William Shakespeare, Othello, circa 1603

Anyone can do a night. The first few weeks following this will be the hardest. Time and time again you will be placed in situations where you are conditioned to have a drink. This might be catching up with old friends, attending work drinks, coming home after work, being depressed, being happy — the list goes on.

For me the toughest time — the time I almost broke - was when I was cooking up a stew. I always drank when I cooked, so I had to fight very strong conditioning every time I picked up a knife to prepare something. On this occasion I lifted a bottle of old wine up to my mouth and almost drank it to see if I could use it in my cooking.

I caught myself just in time, felt angry at the stupidity of it all, and cried out in frustration. I really felt that the whole giving up the drink thing was ridiculous. Surely there was no harm it. It wasn't even drinking. It was bloody stupid, that's what it was.

But I didn't drink it. I felt the symbolism was important.

The first time I was between drinks (for two months at age 25) the thing that broke me was a good friend's wedding. I didn't drink at first. Then someone brought around the champagne. We were in a beautiful room. The bride looked gorgeous Everyone was so happy.

It was just wrong to not drink some champagne to wish my friend the best in her union. It was tradition, it was harmless, it was the right thing to do culturally.

And so I toasted her, and drank my champagne.

With that ended my 8 weeks off the drink experiment. I got pissed that day (yes, it was wonderful) and slid back into old habits. It would be 8 years before I tried again.[18]

Exercise is critical in the first few weeks from a motivational perspective.[19] If you want to feel better off the drink then not abusing yourself with alcohol is only part of it. To get the full benefit (and to make an informed a decision after your trial is over) you really need to take advantage of the additional time and freshness that not drinking provides and make some healthy choices.

You should also use this time to transition to eating as cleanly as you can. With a sound (sober) mind, not punished by

---

[18]   Nigel Marsh, the author of *Forty, Fat and Fired*, suggests that if you can't imagine not having a drink at a wedding then perhaps you have more of a dependency on alcohol than you care to admit. I was so outraged at this in my drinking days that I wrote to him to abuse him. Lovely.

[19]   Assuming of course you don't feel so awful due to withdrawal you can't, in which case you should see your doctor.

hangovers, there is less of an excuse for the nasty late night meals or early morning nightmares. A nutritionist once said that the UK remains a nice little control group reminding the rest of the world of the negative health consequences of a shocking diet, but you don't have to be part of the statistics if you take back control of your time and your mind.

I personally found that I reached levels of fitness that just were not possible when I was getting drunk twice a week. Thanks also to an improved, sober, diet (and less alcohol calories), I also lost weight – over 3 stone (20kg) in 12 months, which is why not drinking for a while is a package of good things and not just the lack of hangovers or bad behaviour.

ACTIONS

1. Keep the faith for the first few weeks, which are the hardest
2. Exercise as much as you can
3. Eat as cleanly as you can

From 3 to 6 months

*The habit of using ardent spirits, by men in office,
has occasioned more injury to the public and
more trouble to me, than all other causes.*

Thomas Jefferson, circa 1800

Everyone is different, but to me, to be honest, I continued to find not drinking difficult even after 3 months. I was still a drinker holding back each time I went out. After all, I was coming (as you probably are) from a background in which drinking was not only expected but was embraced, and, in my case, went to the core of my being.

I was the beer guy. Everyone wanted to talk to me about beer. Everyone wanted to have a beer with me. People sent me beer for free, in the hope I would write about it.[20]

I was also hopelessly Australian (which could just have easily been hopelessly English, or any number of drunken nationalities). Culturally, not only was drinking desirable but it was *offensive* to not have a drink. My people drank every time they got together. Friends. Foes. Family. Strangers. Workmates. Potential clients. Existing clients. Lovers.

I got drunk with the lot of them. And they got drunk with me.

In fact, Australians have been getting drunk ever since our English and Irish forefathers first rolled the kegs of rum off the first fleet back in 1788. And our love of grog goes a whole lot further back than that.[21]

So, yes it was hard. My diary and my exercise helped. Having a defined goal of 12 months helped. Otherwise I would have slipped back into the drunken cycle of work and play so many are familiar with.

The diary gave me some context: how far I had come, the struggles I had had, the patterns I had to watch out for. As it was in the form of a blog comments by strangers who were on their own journey with grog really helped as well.

---

[20] They still do, three years later.
[21] 10,000 years say some. Longer, say others. Pete Brown points out that elephants manage to get pissed on fermented fruit in the jungle and we are a whole lot smarter than they are.

But I kept feeling better, physically and mentally. I looked better, felt better and was more alert. I was happier. People commented on that, which I found amazing. I laughed more.

They do say alcohol is a depressant. But then, who wouldn't laugh more if you were looking better and feeling better.

I still had to be mindful every time I went out. I felt strong physical pangs whenever I was placed in a situation where I would normally have a drink: at lunch, at a meal, when friends drank, and so on. They hit me like a strong emotion (or perhaps a bus), and I had to consciously resist them - which I did, because I wanted to finish my year off the drink.

Pleasingly though I was not desperate for a drink when by myself. I think some lost souls are. Surely they have all the more need to let it go.[22]

Case Study – Bob Hawke

Being a drinker isn't going to bar you from a life in Australian politics, in fact it is considered by many to be a prerequisite.[23] Australia's most colourful Prime Minister – Bob Hawke, was a *huge* drinker, and in fact is most famous among the Australian people for his Guinness Book of Record's world record for beer drinking. That's right, in the 1950s he drank 2.5 pints in 11 seconds!

---

[22]   Richard Feynmen, the famous Nobel prize winning scientist, gave up the drink after he found himself getting drawn into pubs when he walked past even though there was no logical reason for him to be there. He didn't like not being in control of his mind. He still spent time in strip clubs though – sober.

[23]   See http://www.australianbeers.com/culture/politics.htm.

Even though Bob saw his drinking prowess as one of his main positives with the electorate, he voluntarily decided to give up the drink during his period as Prime Minister, which was for 11 years. This was so he could think clearly and properly discharge his duties.

Was he anti-drink? Not at all, in fact if you search for "Bob Hawke Skulling" on YouTube you will see Bob – now in his 80s - playing it up for the camera and downing beers for the benefit of the crowd – he returned to the drink as soon as he got kicked out of office. In one video he is even teaching a young man how to drink faster, all with a cheeky grin on his face.

This is an excellent example of someone – a very bright someone[24] - choosing to spend some time off the drink in order to change their life. Here Bob wanted to free his brain and time in order to think better and be the best Prime Minister he could be. Being hung over or drunk isn't cool when you have to decide if the country is to go to war, after all.[25]

ACTIONS

1.   Do everything in your power to fill in your days with life-giving and stunning activities that you would not have had the time or inclination to do if drunk and hungover
2.   Reinvent yourself, if only for this period in your life

---

[24]   Bob Hawke was a Rhodes Scholar.
[25]   Another famous leader who gave up the booze was George W. Bush. He said that he found it was competing with his energy. Say what you may about the guy, he found the energy to become the most powerful person in the world, and that isn't easy. Maybe being sober helped.

6 to 12 months

A man when drunk is as led by a boy, stumbling and not knowing where he goes, since his soul is moist.

Ephesus, circa 500 BC

After about 6 months it should get much easier. People won't hassle you so much, and by this point, you really won't care. Many observers will be curious about what you are up to, and why you are so chirpy and look so fine. You will be surprised by the number of people who deep down know that they are drinking more than they should. One girl I spoke to – a highly functional lawyer - admitted she was drinking two bottles of wine a night by herself.

Two bottles!

To me, for this slight girl, that's alcoholic territory. At the time I gave up I would feel a bit dusty if I had two beers the night before, and I was twice the size of this girl.

Of course, getting pissed like this gets less and less cool the older you get. Who doesn't like to see a giggling drunk 20 year old? Now picture your mum (once 20 herself) just as drunk and all over the place, collapsing at 2 in the morning in the garden, legs strewn.

It's a nightmare.

A mother of one of my friends always considered herself pretty sophisticated. She would cook nice food and in the French way (or so she thought) she would always have a wine or two at night. Well and good but as the decades passed she became messier and messier and more and more of an embarrassment to her son.

She would get pissed every night, drinking a least a bottle or so.

Not a good look to see your mother pissed that way, slurring her words, face prematurely aged from the drink. When she got a promotion at work and a new title to go with it, she ended up drunkenly ringing a frequent flying club to tell them the good news (she proudly recounted to me days later – also over a drink- how pleased they were for her).

That's pure nuts. This wonderful and very smart lady turned into a pathetic drunk by her late 40s.

But we digress. From 6 to 12 months, things should be getting much easier. The pangs felt in drinking situations should fade. In my case, by the 12 month mark, I could report that the urges, which used to occur every time I was in a social situation, had lessened to once in every 3 months or so.[26]

There is a risk that those feelings of regret and loss felt by not drinking will be replaced by boredom when out with drinkers during a ong binge. I won't lie. Those big nights out you used to have? Unless you are 22, you will quickly find them getting pretty tired pretty fast. You can still participate if you want, but that mind-bending routine of listening to drunken buffoons[27] spit in your face as they guffaw and

---

[26] 3 years in, and I pretty well never feel it. I don't even notice when people are drinking. t doesn't bother me. I don't even notice. This really is proof that you can change the deepest of habits. It amazes me and anyone who knew me. I guess ex-chan smokers must feel the same way.

[27] Sorry, but stick it out a few months and you'll know what I mean.

repeat meaningless stories you have already heard will become less and less appealing as time goes on.

Of course, this realisation doesn't mean your life becomes boring. It's just that you are clearly seeing how you were spending a significant portion of your time for the first time.[28]

The good news is that not drinking lets you do a swap: you exchange those few drunken hours at night (which granted, are fun), with all sorts of cool adventures the next day, when all of your friends are feeling sorry for themselves, drinking caffeinated beverages and eating fattening food.

In fact, if you don't start filling up your newly freed time with cool adventures then chances are your life *will be* boring, and it might be best for everyone if you went back on the drink.....

ACTIONS

1. Enjoy how you are feeling
2. As you start to gain perspective, run with it
3. Become the healthiest you can be without the constant interruption of boozing

---

[28] This can be scary for some – others never acknowledge it, preferring to live in denial. We all do it at some time or another.

CLEAR THINKING

Happy day, when, all appetites controlled, all
poisons subdued, all matter subjected, **mind***,*
all conquering **mind***, shall live and move, the*
monarch of the world. Glorious consummation!
Hail fall of Fury! Reign of Reason, all hail!

Abraham Lincoln speaking about getting
off the drink, February 22, 1842

Seeing drunken nights out for what they really are is just the beginning. As time goes on you will gain more and more perspective on more and more aspects of your life. Eventually, you will gain such insight, and your mind will become so sharp that you will become what I referred to earlier as a Clear Thinker.

Clear Thinking is the ability to see the world and your place in it as it really is, to think about changes you would like made, and making them.

This all sounds like hippy stuff, and believe you me I would have been the most ferocious critic out there before I went through this myself. And to be honest, there are undoubtedly many ways to get to this point: meditation, chatting with whoever looms large in your spiritual paradigm, years of therapy – who knows what other paths there are.

But for people who have let the grog monster grab them by the tail, I am 100 percent confident that breaking that pattern and letting your mind and soul recover for a good while can give you an opportunity to ask some of the bigger questions, and make real changes to your life as a result.

The truth is that when you are in a routine, especially one that involves drinking too much, it is extremely difficult to see the woods for the trees. Life becomes a blurred cycle of going out, getting drunk, getting home, feeling tired, thinking about going out and then going out again. Add a soul destroying job that you drink to recover from, and it takes a superhuman effort to work out what you need to do to stop hurting yourself; to make your life – your day-to-day life – better for you.

Being off the grog for a while can help you do this.

No part of your life should be immune from consideration. But how you spend the bulk of your precious time – doing your job – should be a prime candidate for analysis. What the outcome of the increased perspective will be will naturally depend on your circumstances and your desires. But at least you will have considered it.

Many people who turn to drink for relief are trapped in jobs that suck the life out of them, either through physical demands (80 hour weeks), stress (which can result in all sorts of health problems) or perhaps worst of all, the slow boil of mind numbing tedium.

Why do they stay? Well, that's it, they have never really thought about it. It is just the way it is. They haven't considered things like whether they can reduce their cost base to remove the dependency on their higher income,[29] whether they can in time work part time or get a more fulfilling job, whether they can start up an online business and so on.

In my case, I found that I wanted to make a change, even though I was very well remunerated as a Partner in a large law firm, and wasn't independently wealthy. Previously I never really entertained the thought due to the momentum that built up over 10 years and a high amount of debt.

Your self audit need not lead to downsizing. You may determine you want to be a dynamo at work (or at another workplace) and decide to move to New York and use your time and energy to form the next Google.

Of course, awareness does not mean easy answers. Not drinking does not equate to the waving of a magic wand. Making changes in your life can take a long time, sometimes years, depending on their nature.[30]

I used my newfound clarity to determine that I wanted to head in a different, less materialistic and more time rich direction. Three years (and much effort) later I was able to do so, and left the firm to become a children's book author on the Gold Coast hinterland.[31] The detail of how I did this or what I did is not important. The main point is that not drinking helped give me the perspective I needed to work out what

---

[29] For example, some choose to sell the damn house and investment properties bought with future earnings (debt!) and buy something they can afford that doesn't trap them into 30 years of eyeball popping pain.

[30] Other changes can be made in an instant.

[31] See www.davidjdownie.com.

I really wanted to be doing with my time, and the time and smarts necessary to implement that change.[32]

In your case, the direction you wish to take is unlikely to reveal itself quickly. At the moment you are probably aware things aren't quite right. Listen to yourself! They aren't. Going between drinks for a while will make it easier for you to sort yourself out, to listen to your body and your inner self. A drunken routine makes it almost impossible to hear what they have to say, and what they have to say is critical to your health and wellbeing.

Clearly this self awareness can extend to whether or not you are in a happy place in your relationship. If all you share with your partner is getting drunk and subsequent relations you might think about whether or not that's really all you want.[33] It may be you have less in common than you thought.

Thankfully, it is more likely that your relationship will improve off the drink. I found (to my surprise) that I was far less snappy. Not drinking makes you a more even tempered person, and gives you more (quality) time together to do awesome things with your partner.[34]

Your health too can come under the spotlight away from the booze. Without trying, you should lose weight and become fitter just by virtue of your body not having to process the demon drink. The sober perspective should let you see some objectivity about where you are healthwise.[35] You can

---

[32] For example, I wrote and published 6 books before I left work. Try doing that hung over!

[33] Having said that it does sound pretty good.

[34] Do they like doing awesome things that don't involve drink? Have you ever asked?

[35] A doctor can also help you here. Ever had a full checkup? You aren't 20 any more, God knows.....

then take advantage of this increased strength and vitality, as well as an abundance of new time, to engage in fantastically healthy activities if that takes your fancy.[36]

Finally, you will be able to ask yourself, apart from your income producing activities, relationship and health, how you want to spend the rest of the time that makes up the day-to-day existence of your life. You've replaced, at least for the moment, the night for the day. You can do whatever you want to do, and be whoever you want to be. New skills are there for the learning. You can get really good at something crazy; live those long forgotten childhood fantasies. In fact, while your mates remain trapped in the cycle of massive pint consumption as they moan about everything and tell tired jokes you've been able to...... what? Insert anything you bloody like! Rock climbing? Abseiling? Travel? Languages? Volunteering? You've got all the time and freshness in the world to do it (plus the beer money you've saved).

It will be awesome.

Whatever you end up doing with different aspects of your life, Clear Thinking gives you the ability to do it deliberately and intentionally. It doesn't come after one day off the drink, or even after one week or one month. It really does take months – over 6 in my case, but can give you a chance to re-evaluate and reset the direction of your entire life.

Who knows where you will end up?

---

[36] You might even give up TV. I've replaced mine with a fireplace and bush sounds.

ACTIONS

1. Use your amazing new found clarity about yourself (including your job and those around you) to redesign your life so it is everything you could ever want it to be
2. Spend your new time and energy implementing this change

BACK ON
THE DRINK

Ah, good ol' trustworthy beer.
My love for you will never die.

Homer Simpson

Of course, this book is about being *between* drinks. It's an opportunity to re-evaluate how you want to live your life in a deep way after gaining true perspective.

But what do you do when your allotted not drinking time is up? Unquestionably, a life well lived can involve drink. A beautiful glass of wine, or two, with a meal or a cold beer after mowing the lawn surely is something to enjoy, and can even improve aspects of your health according to a number of studies.

The question is whether or not you actually drink like that. Clearly you didn't exercise such restraint before taking the time of the booze or you wouldn't have been getting drunk so often. You most likely have – if you are honest – restraint issues with alcohol caused by lots of things including your dodgy mates, societal expectations, learned behaviour, your stressful job and so on.[37]

So don't kid yourself. It is a very slippery slope.

---

[37] Or maybe it's just me.

So, with that as background, the experience you have had off the drink, and the perspective you have gained during this period, the big questions for you to consider when pondering next steps is..... *whether or not your life, on balance, is better off the drink than on.*

Is it? Think back to when you decided to buy this book. Is your life better now than it was then, looking at it as a whole?

Of course there can be a downside to not drinking. Drinking is awesome. But the upside can be more awesome, and completely life changing, as hopefully you have seen or at least sensed during your period of abstinence.

There is no right or wrong answer. I cannot tell you. I do not want to tell you. It depends entirely on you, how drink fits into your life, and how you derive pleasure in life.

For me, I had little doubt after my 12 months off the drink that, on balance, my life was much better not drinking. This was the right decision for me – my life was all the richer for it, and continues to amaze three years later.[38] But for you? Maybe not. It depends.

My mother has an excellent relationship with the drink, and it would be cruel and unnecessary (and probably unhealthy) to deprive her of the odd tipple. But most of my mates...... I think they would be better off without it, to be honest. Or drinking moderately, if they can. But who do you know that actually does that? I don't know anyone (apart from my mother). Australia, like the UK and America, is full of binge

---

[38] Especially that I have now implemented my plan and have a completely different life to the booze drenched one I had – and the lack of booze is the least of the differences. In a sense my new post-booze life is just beginning.

drinkers who aren't even aware they are partaking. I don't think moderation is in their vocabulary.[39]

In any event, nobody can answer that question but you, preferably after you have become a Clear Thinker and obtained all the perspective in the world.

Is your life, on balance, better without drinking?

Whatever your decision, at least you will have made an informed one.

---

[39] I thought it was in mine. But looking back, it was anything but.

THIRSTY FOR MORE?

Join me at www.betweendrinksblog.com where you can share your story and be inspired by other Clear Thinkers who are changing their lives, between drinks.

In terms of other books, when the student is ready, the master will appear. What you are ready for, and which masters will appear, will depend entirely on you. That is what (clear) thinking is about!

In my case, I was ready for a downshift, but then I had gone through the corporate ringer for almost 20 years. You may be gearing up to become a software billionaire, or the world's greatest curry chef.

Either way, these are some of the books that have influenced me on my journey. You will notice none of them deal with giving up the grog. I haven't found anyone who thinks about grog the way I do.

Mind Over Medicine: Scientific Proof You
Can Heal Yourself by Lisa Rankin

No, she isn't a nutter, she's a doctor taking a big picture approach. Your health and vitality problems may have more to do with your dysfunctional relationship or soul destroying job than anything else. The solution? Write your own prescription. Sign me up.

The Four Hour Work Week by Tim Ferris

Many people know this book and the general conclusion is that this guy's a bullshitter. I disagree. I think he really challenges you to think outside the box, and reject the boring path the system has in store for you. Not for those without spine. Read this one over and over as most don't get it at first.

Choosing Simplicity: Real People Finding Peace and Fulfillment in a Complex World by Linda Breen Pierce

Linda does a great job here examining real life examples of people who have made changes in their lives after a period of reflection.

www.ingramcontent.com/pod-product-compliance
Lightning Source LLC
Chambersburg PA
CBHW072021290326
41934CB00009BA/2154